Leaf Your Weight Behind

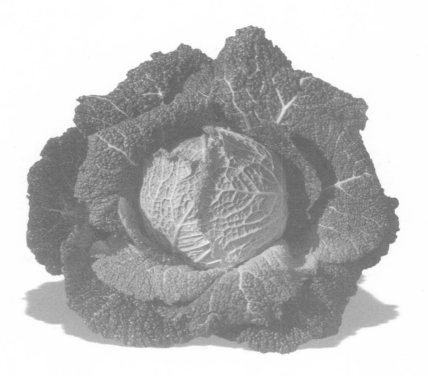

Leaf Your Weight Behind

A plan for life:
losing the weight and keeping it off forever!

Nancy Barnes & Marina Volynets

Whenever starting a new diet, we recommend that you consult your physician first. The "Leaf Your Weight Behind" program in no way claims to heal or eliminate particular health problems.

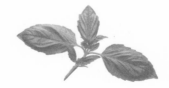

This book is dedicated to our children: Carrie, Katie, and Anna Claire, and to their children after them that they will take the challenge to eat healthy and to live holy.

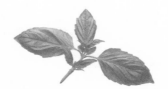

All things are lawful for me, but not all things are profitable. All things are lawful for me, but I will not be mastered by anything.

1 Corinthians 6:12
(NASB)

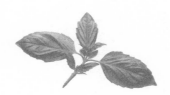

Contents

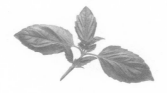

As an orthopedic surgeon, I frequently see patients that suffer with orthopedic problems as a result of excess weight. Many of these patients are at wits end because they feel they have tried everything to lose weight.

I can gladly recommend Leaf Your Weight Behind to them because it is a sensible, healthy plan that works. It worked for me! I lost 25 pounds and I didn't even have time to exercise. The benefits of this program combined with exercise will produce great results. I believe this is the program that people are looking for to give them a healthy lifestyle.

I enthusiastically recommend it to my patients and enthusiastically recommend it to you!

—Dr. Bill Barnes
Piedmont Sports Medicine Clinic
Macon, Georgia

Introduction

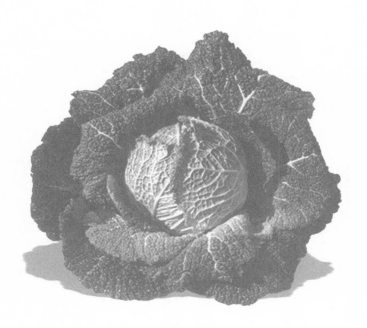

Our lives have been forever enhanced since Vadim and Marina Volynets came to live with us two years ago. Natives of Kiev, Ukraine, the Volynets came to the United States to perform with their symphony orchestra and once here, they decided to stay. Imagine the impact of forsaking all for a new life in America. Having only their musical instruments and one suitcase of clothing, month by month they stayed with different families from First Presbyterian Church, Macon, Georgia, waiting and hoping for their work permit to come so they could perform music again.

Only a short while after Vadim and Marina came to live in our home did we tell them they never had to move again and could stay with us as long as they needed. Not only are they magnificent musicians and incredible people, but they are monumental in their knowledge of health and nutrition. Marina not only performed with several symphony orchestras, but also was trained as a chef in her native country. As Marina and I cooked together in my home, something *magical* happened! We often talk about the unusual circumstances that brought us together—to meet, to live in the same home, to work together in the kitchen. We are amazed that our paths crossed in such a way. After all, if they hadn't, we wouldn't have created truly delicious and nutritious meals that enabled us to lose weight. We had so much fun doing it! **YOU WILL TOO!**

Marina had gained 20 pounds in the first three months of living in the United States and eating the "Great American Diet." An extra 20 pounds had jumped on me from somewhere. I hadn't figured out where, because I was a low-fat maniac. I was a devoted fat gram counter. Truly we were both very frustrated. We became determined to create meals for our family that would put us all on the road to better health. This is not just about losing weight. It's about quality of life! I really believe that most folks out there are just like us—they want to be **HAPPY** and **HEALTHY** They want to cook the right foods for themselves and their families.

We combined Marina's marvelous salads and my study of carbohydrates (carbs) and how they affect the body to create a menu of meals that could keep us healthy and help us lose weight at the same time. We think it can help you, too!

Even if you don't need to lose weight, this book will equip you with some great recipes and information for a healthier lifestyle. I can take no credit for the recipes; they are the creations of Chef Marina! Neither can I take credit for the information on carbohydrates. I've just gleaned information from various sources and passed it along to you. Remember: We do not claim to be experts! This book is a response to people who kept clamoring for us to write this information down for them. So here it is—an easy and simple guide of menus and recipes, along with a carbohydrate counter to help you *Leaf Your Weight Behind.*

This book is written to give you **hope**—hope that you can and will lose that weight you've been trying to get off for years and will keep it off for the rest of your life! **OUR PLAN IS NOT A DIET** It is a guide to help you develop a lifestyle of healthy eating habits. You will lose weight, absolutely! You will also feel great! When you put the right foods into your body, you will have more energy and fewer health problems, and your entire mental well-being will improve! Unlike following a diet, following our plan will not make you feel deprived, depressed, or defeated!

Leaf Your Weight Behind is about a lifestyle of eating the foods that give us life—leaves, including cabbage leaves, spinach leaves, lettuce leaves, beet leaves, celery leaves, etc. It's about mainly eating "live" raw vegetables and fruits, not cooked ones. These fresh whole foods contain the vitamins and minerals essential to healthy living. Doesn't sound very a "peeling" to you? How would you like to lose 15 to 20 pounds in the next two or three months and **ENJOY DOING IT?**

What in the world am I talking about? Why write another book on salads and vegetables when there are an abundance out there already? Because **OUR PLAN WORKS** and people are desperate for a simple plan that will **SHOW THEM HOW** and **GIVE THEM HOPE**. Many people are just like I was: not knowing whether to count fat grams or calories, eat only protein, or go on a liquid diet—**HELP!** People want help, and everyone with whom we share this plan gets so excited about it. Why? Because it is easy and it works! They lose weight when they follow our plan. You will lose weight, too. You will also develop a healthy lifestyle that will enable you to **KEEP THE WEIGHT OFF FOREVER!**

After I lost 20 pounds, people kept asking me how I did it. Marina lost 15 pounds. My husband lost 20, and my daughter lost 15. My sister-in-law lost 25 pounds and is still losing. I recently visited my brother and shared the plan with him and his wife. I cooked for them the recipes from our book during the four days I was there. His wife lost 3 pounds in just four days! (My brother lost only 1 because he cheated and didn't do what I told him!) Our good friends, Dr. Ken and Terri Harper, lost 25 and 15 pounds, respectively. Terri is so excited about our plan that she has shared it with more than 25 people, and all of them who have followed the plan have lost weight. **THIS IS IT! THIS PLAN WORKS!** This plan may be the lifestyle solution for which you have been looking and it is so easy! I've had so many people tell me that after trying every diet out there, this plan is the one that really makes sense and works for them.

—Nancy Barnes

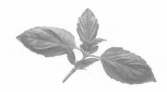

How Does the Plan Work?

I read an article in our local Macon paper that stated that our low-fat, high-carbohydrate diets have been making Americans fatter and sicker. Dr. Barry Sears states in "Zone Perfect Meals in Minutes" that today we are eating less fat than in any other time in history, yet we have become the fattest people on the face of the earth! Dr. Everett Koop called **OBESITY** the greatest public health crisis currently facing our nation. Go to the mall and sit and watch people. Have you ever seen so many chubby people in your life? Old ladies, old men, teenagers, and small children are lining up at the fast food places and getting **fatter** and **fatter** as they eat a diet bulging with excess carbohydrates.

Now our book is neither scientific or academic. It is a practical guide to help you with your battle against the bulge. But it is important that you understand why a low-fat, high-carbohydrate diet can make you fat.

Dr. Sears says that the average American will eat the carbohydrate equivalent of **2 cups of sugar** each day. What does that mean? It means that most people would never eat four chocolate candy bars at a time but would have no problem eating eight ounces of pasta, which has the same amount of carbohydrates. As Dr. Sears emphasizes, your stomach can't tell the difference.

The more carbohydrates you eat, the more insulin your body produces. Sears explains that insulin is a storage hormone whose function is to push incoming calories into cells. Excess carbohydrates that can't be stored are immediately converted to fat. Insulin drives this newly converted fat into fat cells for storage. Therefore, the more insulin you produce, the fatter you become. The fatter you become, the more you endanger your health.

Sears refers to carbohydrates as **DRUGS.** Consumption of too many will give rise to toxic side effects such as overproduction of insulin, which can be really dangerous. You can become **ADDICTED** to carbohydrates and literally crave and be dependent upon the false sense of satisfaction they give! Again, when you ingest more carbohydrates than your body needs, your body will store them as fat. This is the reason a low-fat, high-carbohydrate diet can *keep us from losing weight* and can endanger our health.

How healthy is your routine? Consider a typical American breakfast on the go—a bagel and a glass of orange juice. Unfortunately, this is among the worst choices for breakfast. **"Why? Why? Why?"** you scream! You thought you were being *so good, so healthy, so lowfat!* You even used diet margarine. You only had 3 grams of fat instead of 20 grams had you eaten bacon and eggs. *This plan is not about fat, which does not raise your insulin level! This plan is about Carbohydrates—rapid inducers of insulin!* With bacon and eggs you have only 2 carbohydrates. A bagel and OJ breakfast contain 75 grams of carbohydrates!

"It can't be!" you moan in anguish. Unfortunately, all the fat-free pretzels, fat-free cookies, fat-free tortilla chips, and fat-free salad dressings you dutifully consume are *loaded with carbohydrates.* After hearing about our plan, people always ask me, "What about the fat?" Don't worry! You will not be consuming unlimited fat. As you limit your carbohydrate intake, you will automatically trim your fat intake because many fat-laden foods are also carbohydrate-dense.

Think of some of the most obese people groups in the world and I guarantee you that their diet is high in carbohydrates. It doesn't matter if it is brown rice and buckwheat or brownies and bagels. Remember: Your stomach can't tell the difference. The more carbohydrates you consume, the more insulin you produce. The more insulin you produce, the more fat you store.

I remember when I was in the no meat, complex carbohydrate craze. We had oat groats for breakfast, kasha for lunch, and buckwheat for supper. When my family started saying "Neigh" instead of "No" and we were getting stocky like horses, I decided that all that grain was making us fat. Luckily for us, it was near that time when Marina and Vadim moved in with us and helped us get on the right track.

Basically our plan is this: Keep your carbohydrate intake to **60 grams** or less per day and you will lose weight. **Did you hear me?** Eat **60 grams** of carbohydrates a day and you **WILL** lose weight!! That's it. That's all. Isn't that **SIMPLE?** You are not counting calories. You are not counting fat grams. You are simply counting carbohydrates. This is not a high protein, no carbohydrate diet. This is a <u>normal protein, low carbohydrate lifestyle.</u>

Counting carbohydrates is different and easier that counting calories. It is very important for you to chart your progress and to gain an awareness of every carb that enters your body. We have included a carbohydrate counter to assist you. Record all the food you eat and the number of carbohydrates contained in each food. This is especially critical after you complete the 2-week menu plan. You will be on your own, although repeating the menus is a guaranteed method for keeping to the 60 carbs limit. (Most of the carbohydrate counts we include are taken from the package. In all other cases we utilized Dr. Art Ulene's book *Nutrition Fact Desk Reference*.)

Our 2-week menu does the work for you. You won't have to worry about what you are going to prepare for dinner. After two weeks, you will definitely have lost weight. Make any substitutions you desire, but make sure you stay at 60 carbs daily. If you do not like some of the cheeses suggested, substitute a hard cheese, not a processed cheese.

Remember: <u>Count carbohydrates,</u> not fat and not calories. Also remember that you want to keep your car- bohydrate intake to **60 grams** daily. (You may need to adjust that figure more or less to suit you.) If you follow the plan but do not lose weight fast enough, you may choose to not include snacks in your daily routine or to not eat toast at breakfast. Also, you can double up on salad portions and omit cooked vegetables if they don't interest you.

On the other hand, some people need to eat more than 60 carbohydrates daily. If you are fatigued and have difficulty concentrating, enjoy four snacks each day instead of only two. You might enjoy half an apple and cheddar cheese, celery with peanut butter, half a banana with a small handful of almonds, or and extra 1/2 cup of strawberries. As with any dietary change, your body will initially struggle with our plan. The absence of processed junk food and all sugar may be quite a shock to your system. Usually the tired feeling passes in just a few days as your body adjusts to your consuming luscious, live, fruits and vegetables. It is important that you drink eight glasses of water each day. If you have any concerns, consult your doctor.

Following the plan successfully requires that you change the way you think about food. Following are a few examples of how you will need to change your mindset.

- Let's say you snack on carrots all day long. Isn't that healthy? One medium carrot contains 5 grams of carbohydrates. If you eat six of these carrots, you've already consumed half of your daily allotment of 60 carbs.

- I hate skim milk in my coffee. It's so thin and weak. Did you realize that skim milk contains more carbs than cream? I now use cream and **ENJOY** it so much more.

- You mean that I would be better off eating two crackers with 2 teaspoons of natural peanut butter than 1/2 cup pretzels? The two peanut butter crackers contain 7 carbs while just 1 ounce of pretzels (only a small handful) contain 21 grams of carbohydrates!

- What about 1/2 cup of low fat frozen yogurt verses 1/2 cup vanilla ice cream? "Ice cream is the drug of choice?" *you gasp incredulously!* Read the facts and weep. 1/2 cup of vanilla ice cream contains 15 carbs; 1/2 cup of low-fat yogurt contains 24 carbs. Which one would you rather have?

- Low-fat chips? That's right—22 carbs in just one ounce! That's only about 15 chips.

- Should we talk about beverages? A can of cola contains 38 carbs. Eight ounces of orange juice contain 30 carbs, apple juice 28, and grape juice 40.

When I made discoveries such as these, I began to understand why I couldn't lose weight. I opened my pantry and looked at all the low-fat foods that were **high in carbohydrate misery** and I wept! See for yourself. Read the statistics on all the ready-to-eat cereals in your pantry. Check the carbs on all the fat-free salad dressings in your refrigerator. You will be shocked!

Stay away from all kinds of pasta, cereals, granola, breads, cakes, and cookies unless you plan to count those in your 60 grams per day. I eat one slice of whole wheat toast with my egg in the morning. It contains 14 grams of carbs. Therefore, I have 45 grams left for the rest of the day. I choose meals carefully and "spend" those remaining carbs in the most satisfying way. For example, if I have a special dinner or party planned for the evening, I consume no carbs at breakfast or at lunch so I can enjoy all 60 carbs at dinner!

Avoid candy, dried fruits, fruit juices, frozen yogurt, sherbet, pastries, carbonated drinks (diet drinks are acceptable but not encouraged) beer, and ale. You can occasionally eat fruits and vegetables that are high in carbohydrates. These include bananas, mangoes, corn, potatoes, carrots, lima beans, dried beans, and peas.

Why no fruit juices? Fruit juices are extremely dense in carbohydrates. When you drink fruit juice, you don't get the satisfaction of chewing or crunching, and you consume nearly half of the total carbs allowed for the entire day! I'd rather eat my carbs than drink them. So, instead of drinking juices, I drink filtered water and herbal teas. I also have a glass of dry red wine with dinner.

Did those of you who are addicted to sodas scream when you read in the previous list that you consume 38 grams of carbohydrates when you drink one can of cola? Give them up. There are nearly 12 teaspoons of sugar in each can. What about diet sodas? Although diet sodas do not contain carbs, they are not necessarily a good beverage choice. Aspartame, Equal, and Nutrasweet used in diet drinks and many low-fat foods deplete the body's supply of chromium, a mineral which plays a crucial role in sugar metabolism. According to Ann Gittleman in her book *Get the Sugar Out*, insufficient chromium also leads to insulin inefficiency, which in turn leads to greater insulin resistance. Ms. Gittleman states that even though artificial sweeteners are advertised as sugar alternatives, dextrose, a sugar, is an ingredient in of each of them. She says studies have shown that the use of aspartame may actually increase your sugar and carbohydrate cravings! So now I know why a candy bar and diet cola taste so good together.

Let's talk about sugar. Notice that none of our recipes include sugar and no desserts are listed. We are trying to get the sugar out of your system so you won't crave the carbohydrates. We realize that life without sugar is next to impossible for some, but try it for two weeks. You will feel so much better and look leaner, too. If you must have sugar in your coffee, use pure crystalline fructose, a fruit sugar made from corn. Fructose contains carbohydrates but only slightly stimulates insulin, causing less of a rise and fall in blood sugar levels. Avoid liquid fructose, or corn syrup.

Check your labels. You will learn that sugar is added to food you never dreamed would have it—canned tomatoes, beans, soups, low fat salad dressings, cocktail sauce, catsup to list a few. Any sweetener dramatically increases the carbohydrate content of food. Be familiar with some of the "hidden" names of sugar. Since the list of terms for hidden sugar is huge, I will list a few.

Table 1

barley malt	corn sugar	mannitol
beet sugar	dextrose	maple syrup
blackstrap molasses	dulcitol	molasses
brown sugar	fructose	polydextrose
cane sugar	fruit juice	sorbitol
cane syrup	fruit sugar	sorbo
caramel coloring	glucose	sorghum
caramel flavoring	grape sugar	whey
caramel malt	honey	xylitol
	lactose	
	malt	
	maltose	

Eat Your Vegetables!

Many of you have lost weight on a high-protein, no carbohydrate diet only to gain it all back as soon as you added carbohydrates. We were meant to eat fresh fruits and vegetables. The best foods are fresh, raw, natural foods because they give us life and vital energy. Our plan recommends eating raw vegetable salads because they contain the most vitamins and minerals. Cooking and canning kill the real energy of fruits and vegetables. You will notice that we have very few cooked vegetables in our menus, only a few that are steamed vegetables that still have a "crunch." In our house we don't cook many vegetables. We occasionally have potatoes. We believe that raw, fresh vegetable salads will benefit you the most.

Many of you might be thinking as I did—*"But I hate vegetables!"* Now, I have an entirely different attitude. I **devour** our fresh salads! They are so delicious and satisfying. Even my children, who never wanted the puny lettuce salads I used to fix, enjoy our salads. They eat all the salads and ask for seconds! It's so different from the way we lived before. I often didn't want to cook because I was sick of preparing pasta all the time. I did what all young mothers do when they don't want to cook—eat fast food! It's easy to get in a fast food rut.

But again, **the basic truth**—we were meant to eat fresh fruits and vegetables. We need them for essential nutrition and to add interest to our meals. Admit it. If you had to eat only eggs, cheese, and meat all the time or even for two weeks, wouldn't you be sick? That's why you are going to be **crazy** about our plan. This is going to be so exciting for you. This works and **will work for you!**

Notice in the menus that we suggest "Cabbage Leaf Sandwiches" for lunch. Let me explain why eating cabbage is fundamental to *Leaf Your Weight Behind.* Cabbage is an unbelievably healthy vegetable with amazing properties. It kills bacteria and viruses; prevents cancer, particularly of the colon; heals ulcers; and stimulates the immune system.

According to Dr. James and Phyllis Balch in *Prescription for Cooking and Dietary Wellness*, eating cabbage once a week may reduce your chances of colon cancer by 60%. (Eating it more frequently is likely to boost its anti-cancer potency.) These authors cite conclusive studies. Saxon-Graham, Ph.D., and his colleagues in Buffalo, New York, found that people who never ate cabbage were three times more likely to develop colon cancer. In Japan in 1986, people who consumed cabbage had the lowest death rate from all cancers! Balch and Balch quote the *American Medical Journal* as saying that "cabbage is therapeutically effective in conditions of scurvy, diseases of the eyes, gout, rheumatism (arthritis), pyorrhea, asthma, tuberculosis, cancer, and gangrene." It is excellent as a vitalizing agent and a blood purifier.

These healing capabilities, however, are present only in raw cabbage. Cooking destroys them. The chlorophyll in raw cabbage helps to prevent anemia. The high levels of vitamin A aid in tissue rejuvenation. The sulfur helps fight infection and protects the skin from eczema and other rashes.

Do you eat a lot of bread? My family has always used bread as a "shover" at meals, pushing our food with it. Vadim and Marina Volynets taught our family to eat folded cabbage leaves at meals instead of bread. The cabbage is very satisfying, helps to fill us up, and is quite tasty. Marina also encouraged me to fill a cabbage leaf with whatever I wanted—Canadian bacon, turkey, chopped liver, ham, sautéed tofu, tuna fish, cheese, sprouts, chopped olives—then fold over the leaf and secure with a toothpick. **This became an instant hit!** My husband started taking cabbage leaf sandwiches to work. My daughters wanted them packed in their lunches. I carried a sandwich with me wherever I went in case I got hungry. One day in the beauty salon several women stood around me to see my cabbage leaf sandwich. When I explained to them the benefits of substituting cabbage for bread, they became excited and began to include cabbage leaf sandwiches in their diets.

So don't be surprised if someday when you come to Macon, Georgia there is a sign posted on the outskirts of the city limits:

Welcome to Macon, Georgia
"Home of the Cabbage Leaf Sandwich"

When you think about it, "Leaf Your Weight Behind" was born from the leaf of a cabbage!

Speaking of leaves, let's talk about the leafiest meal— the salad! The salads included in this guide easily feed a family of four. You may need to double or half them to suit your needs. Also, we didn't count the carbs in the salad dressings because our recipes only contain a trace per tablespoon. Don't use more than a tablespoon.

We like to add sprouts to every salad and we grow our own. Wheat sprouts add protein, unbelievable amounts of vitamins and minerals. They are low in carbohydrates. We didn't include sprouts in our recipes because some people are afraid of them. We do think you will use them if you know how. Don't think you can do it? I used to think the same, but it is so easy! Use the following directions and you can enjoy fresh sprouts in your home, too!

Purchase 1 pound of organically grown wheat berries. (That's what they call plain ol' wheat—wheat berries.) Or, you can purchase any other seed that you want (ex: wheat berries, alfalfa, mung beans, cabbage). We use wheat because I have 50 pounds of wheat left over from when I was on the "complex carbohydrate" diet that made us all "stocky."

Buy some plastic screen from the local hardware store. (I didn't even know that such a thing existed!) Clean a wide-mouthed jar and cut an 8" square to fit over the top. Before going to bed, put 1/3 cup wheat or other seed in the jar. Fill the jar with warm, filtered water. Place the screen over the jar mouth and secure with a heavy rubber band (ex: the type that holds together broccoli stalks). The next morning, with the screen snugly secured, turn the jar upside down and allow the water to drain. Rinse the seed by refilling the jar with warm water, then draining as before. Place the drained jar of seed in a dark place in the kitchen. Repeat the process for two or three days. Wheat sprouts will be ready for use when they are about 1/8 inch long; alfalfa sprouts need to be about

1 inch long. When the sprouts are the right length, rinse them, pat them dry, and refrigerate in a plastic container. That usually makes enough fresh sprouts for two days!

Recommendations and Helpful Hints

- Before starting this plan, consult your doctor. It may not be what you need if you have particular health problems. Take your copy of the book and leave it with your doctor. I wouldn't be surprised if he or she chooses to follow our plan, too!

- Drink eight 8-ounce glasses of filtered water each day. To lose weight, drink 8 ounces of water (no ice) 15 minutes *before* you eat. Do not drink water with your meal. Oriental folk healers say drinking water with your meal drowns and dilutes the effectiveness of digestive juices, thus impairing the assimilation of essential nutrients. Wait 1 hour after your meal before drinking any beverages, especially if you have eaten meat.

- You may include herbal teas as part of a day's water requirement. Buy teas in bags or loose at grocery or nutrition stores. We buy loose herbs such as peppermint, spearmint, hibicious leaves, lemon balm. You can use herbs individually or mixed. Peppermint and hibicious leaves are a good combination. Also, Peppermint is a "relaxing" herb so it helps with stress. Be creative!

- Grow your own herbs. I purchased basil, dill, chives, and parsley at a local nursery and replanted them. We now have several herbs growing in pots on the back porch. We use them in everything we cook. Tending the herbs is easy! I know that if I can do it, you can because I'm the kind of person who kills even silk plants.

- To deal with hunger between meals, take two chromium picolinate tablets in mid-morning and mid-afternoon. Remember: Chromium plays a crucial role in sugar metabolism and it helps with sugar cravings. And, once you begin to eat the meals in the menu, your stomach will shrink and you won't feel so hungry.

- Always keep a low-carb snack with you. This little bit of preparation can help you resist the temptation to pull into a convenience store or fast food place when you feel hungry or have cravings.

- If you must eat fast food, choose only foods with low carbohydrate content. If you crave a hamburger, eat only one side of the bun, thus reducing carbohydrate grams from 30 to 15.

- Beware of salad dressings. The low-fat varieties often contain sugar and have 10 or more grams of carbohydrates per tablespoon. Regular Italian dressing has less than 1 carb per tablespoon!

• Check all food labels to determine the number of carbohydrates in each serving. The FDA has made it easy for us by requiring that nutritional information be listed on all packaged foods. You can easily see how many carbohydrates are in a serving of food, not the entire package.

• Bacon and Canadian bacon are optional at breakfast. You may wish to avoid them because they contain nitrates. Use fresh sausage containing no preservatives if possible. You might use leftover pork tenderloin, sliced and sautéed with eggs. Fresh and natural food is always preferred.

• When I buy bacon, I choose the precooked, frozen variety that can be warmed in the microwave.

• When buying red or white cabbage, choose heads that are oval in shape. Leaves are easier to peel off an oval head than a round head.

• If you don't like cabbage, use Romaine lettuce, spinach leaves, or any other green leaf that is large enough to substitute for bread.

• Use a variety of cabbage for your salads and sandwiches. Napa, bok choy, and red and white cabbage all contain anti-cancer chemicals.

- Keep a plastic bag filled with cabbage leaves in the refrigerator. If you don't time to make a cabbage sandwich, take a couple of leaves in a plastic bag for use with a fast food sandwich. For example, buy a roast beef or deli turkey or roasted chicken sandwich, and throw away the bun and put the meat inside the cabbage leaf!

- Of course any salad from fast food places will be fine *if* it is fresh. Unfortunately, the salads sometimes sit for two or three days and might be a little brown or wilted. Always check the age of the salad before you order it. if you eat the croutons or crackers you must count those in your daily total of 60 carbs. Don't use more than a tablespoon of salad dressing. Those goodies can add unwanted carbs in a hurry!

- Watch out for catsup! It contains 4 carbs per tablespoon. If you use any condiment; count it!

- Realize that wine is a suggestion, not a requirement, on the menus. I just think it's cool that dry wine could be considered healthy and doesn't have any carbs. Cheers!

- Where do we buy the products we use? At our local Kroger grocery store. We've found that the health food section at Kroger is fabulous! We don't have to spend hours shopping because every thing we need—Kroger has. We are particularly please with the large organic produce section. There we can get wonderful organic salad greens such as Romaine Lettuce, mixed greens, red and green leaf lettuce, organic carrots, onions and radishes.

• You may want to invest in a food processor. Ours allows us to create a salad in only a few minutes!

• After you've lost the weight you want to lose, add extra fruit and vegetables to your diet. You no longer have to be so concerned with limiting your carbohydrate intake to 60 grams each day. If you do remain at 60 carbs per day, you'll keep losing weight and become *too* skinny.

• Last, but not least—**Have fun with our plan!** Enjoy eating meals together as a family. Be confident that you are doing the best for yourself and your family as you "Leaf Your Weight Behind!"

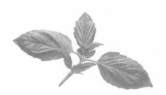

Menus

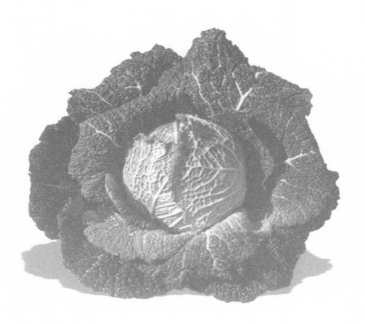

Day 1

Menu Notes

Food: Portion/Size	Carbohydrate Grams

Breakfast

2 eggs	2
1 slice whole wheat toast w/butter	14
2 pieces Canadian bacon (opt.)	0
coffee w/ cream	1
herbal tea	0
	17

Lunch

2 cabbage leaf sandwiches	
(1 oz. deli turkey, Swiss cheese, chopped olives, sprouts)	6
herbal tea	0
	6

Snack

1 oz. cashews	8

Dinner

lemon-caper turkey	2
red leaf lettuce salad	8
green beans almondine	7
dry white or red wine	0
	17

Snack

1 c. sliced strawberries	10
Total	58

Day 2

Menu Notes

Food: Portion/Size	Carbohydrate Grams

Breakfast

1 oz. deli turkey or ham w/ melted cheese	0
1/2 grapefruit	14
coffee w/ cream	1
herbal tea	0
	15

Lunch

Greek salad w/ chicken strips	6
herbal tea	0
	6

Snack

1/2 c. strawberries	5

Dinner

kool cat fish fillets	0
1 ear corn	16
avocado-spinach salad	7
dry white or red wine	0
	23

Snack

2 Wasa light rye crisps	10.8
w/ sun-dried tomato-basil spread	

Total 59.8

Day 3

Menu Notes

_____

_____

_____

_____

_____

_____

_____

_____

_____

_____

_____

_____

_____

Food: Portion/Size	Carbohydrate Grams

Breakfast

2 poached eggs	2
1 slice whole wheat toast w/ butter	14
2 slices bacon (opt.)	0
coffee w/ cream	1
herbal tea	0
	17

Lunch

2 cabbage leaf sandwiches	6
(Canadian bacon, pepper jack cheese, chopped olives and sprouts)	
herbal tea	0
	6

Snack

1/2 c. pecans	7.5

Dinner

pork tenderloin medallions	0
1/2 c. herbed potatoes	18
cabbage-turnip salad	3.5
dry white or red wine	0
	21.5

Snack

1 nectarine	8
	Total 60

Day 4

Menu Notes

_____

_____

_____

_____

_____

_____

_____

_____

_____

_____

_____

_____

_____

Food: Portion/Size	Carbohydrate Grams

Breakfast

1 slice whole wheat toast	14
1 TBS. natural peanut butter	3
1/4 banana, sliced	6
coffee w/ cream	1
herbal tea	0
	24

Lunch

chef salad	6
herbal tea	0
	6

Snack

3 Ritz crackers w/ pecan-olive spread	9.5

Dinner

tender baked chicken	0
red cabbage-cucumber salad	8
steamed broccoli w/ picante sauce	8
dry white or red wine	0
	16

Snack

1/2 peach	4.5
	Total 60

Day 5

Menu Notes

....

....

....

....

....

....

....

....

....

....

....

....

....

Food: Portion/Size	Carbohydrate Grams

Breakfast

cheese-onion omelet	3
2 slices Canadian bacon (opt.)	0
1 slice whole wheat toast w/ butter	14
coffee w/ cream	1
herbal tea	0
	18

Lunch

tofu for you	less than 1
6 spears sautéed asparagus	5
herbal tea	0
	5

Snack

1 oz. peanuts	6

Dinner

smothered salmon	5
bok choy-tomato salad	5
grilled eggplant	7
dry white or red wine	0
	17

Snack

1/2 c. blueberries	11
Total	57

Day 6

Menu Notes

....

....

....

....

....

....

....

....

....

....

....

....

....

Food: Portion/Size	Carbohydrate Grams

Breakfast

1 slice whole wheat toast	14
1 oz. deli turkey	0
1 oz. Swiss cheese	0
coffee w/ cream	1
herbal tea	0
	15

Lunch

chicken salad supreme	5
bed of greens	1
herbal tea	0
	6

Snack

1/2 lg. apple	12
1 oz. sharp cheddar cheese	0
	12

Dinner

ocean perch in tomato-herb sauce	11
romaine-spinach salad	5
dry white or red wine	0
	16

Snack

1/2 c. grapes	10

Total 59

Day 7

Menu Notes

Food: Portion/Size	Carbohydrate Grams

Breakfast

2 eggs	2
1/2 small grapefruit	10
2 slices bacon (opt.)	0
coffee w/ cream	1
herbal tea	0
	17

Lunch

2 cabbage leaf sandwiches (1 oz. deli turkey, Swiss cheese, chopped olives, sprouts)	6
herbal tea	0
	6

Snack

1 peach	9

Dinner

spicy baked chicken	0
mushroom-pepper salad	3
1 sm. baked potato	20
dry white or red wine	0
	23

Snack

1 plum	6
	Total 57

Day 8

Menu Notes

Food: Portion/Size	Carbohydrate Grams

Breakfast

2 scrambled eggs	2
2 slices bacon (opt.)	0
1 slice whole wheat toast w/ butter	14
coffee w/ cream	1
herbal tea	0
	17

Lunch

6 oz. smoked salmon	0
1 TBS. capers	1
1 TBS. chopped sweet onion	1
2 slices rye melba toast	10
herbal tea	0
	12

Snack

1 small kiwi	9

Dinner

terrific trout	2
beet top salad	4
1 ear corn	16
dry white or red wine	0
	22

Snack

1 oz. cheese	0
red wine	0
	Total 60

Day 9

Menu Notes

_____

_____

_____

_____

_____

_____

_____

_____

_____

_____

_____

_____

Food: Portion/Size	Carbohydrate Grams

Breakfast

1 slice whole wheat toast	14
1 TBS. natural peanut butter	4
1 tsp. natural fruit spread	3
coffee w/ cream	1
herbal tea	0
	22

Lunch

2 salmon, tuna, or crab cakes	0
tiny tomato toss	4
herbal tea	0
	4

Snack

1 oz. cashews	8

Dinner

sassy soy chicken strips	0
Napa-beet salad	6
1 c. broccoli w/ butter and garlic	7.5
dry white or red wine	0
	13.5

Snack

1/2 c. fresh blackberries	10
	Total 57.5

Day 10

Menu Notes

Food: Portion/Size	Carbohydrate Grams

Breakfast

western omelet	3
2 pieces Canadian bacon (opt.)	0
1 slice whole toast w/ butter	14
coffee w/ cream	1
herbal tea	0
	18

Lunch

2 cabbage leaf sandwiches (tuna, chopped dill pickles, cheese, mayonnaise, sprouts)	6
herbal tea	0
	6

Snack

4 Ritz crackers	8
1 TBS. peanut butter	4
	14

Dinner

boiled shrimp w/ cocktail sauce	2
tomato-cucumber salad	6
cheesy-yellow squash	5
dry white or red wine	0
	13

Snack

1 c. strawberries	10
	Total 59

Day 11

Menu Notes

Food: Portion/Size	Carbohydrate Grams

Breakfast

2 poached eggs	0
2 slices Canadian bacon (opt.)	0
1 slice whole wheat toast w/butter	14
coffee w/ cream	1
herbal tea	0
	15

Lunch

1 c. chicken livers (approx. 5, each wrapped w/ 1/2 piece bacon)	0
Marina's slaw	8
herbal tea	0
	8

Snack

1 oz. cashews	8

Dinner

luscious leg of lamb	2
red cabbage-pepper salad	5
1 sm. baked potato	20
dry white or red wine	0
	27

Snack

1 oz. cheese	0
dry red wine	0
	Total 58

Day 12

Menu Notes

Food: Portion/Size	Carbohydrate Grams

Breakfast

2 scrambled eggs w/ picante sauce	2
2 slices bacon (opt.)	0
1 slice whole wheat toast w/butter	14
coffee w/ cream	1
herbal tea	0
	17

Lunch

baked chicken breast	0
1 sliced tomato	5
(sprinkled w/ feta cheese and balsamic vinegar)	
herbal tea	0
	5

Snack

2 Wasa light rye crisps	10
crab or tuna spread	1.5
	11.5

Dinner

grilled turkey patties	0
mixed greens-black olive salad	6
tomato-mushroom sauté	8
dry white or red wine	0
	14

Snack

1 c. watermelon	11
	Total 58.5

Day 13

Menu Notes

Food: Portion/Size	Carbohydrate Grams

Breakfast

1 slice whole wheat toast	14
1 TBS. peanut butter	4
1 tsp. natural fruit spread	3
coffee w/ cream	1
herbal tea	0
	22

Lunch

2 cabbage leaf sandwiches	6
(deli turkey, Monterey jack cheese, chopped olives, sprouts)	
herbal tea	0
	6

Snack

3/4 cantaloupe	9

Dinner

grilled scallops w/ Mar-Na sauce	0
avocado-parsley salad	8
1 c. steamed cauliflower w/ cheese	5
dry white or red wine	0
	13

Snack

1 peach	9
	Total 59

Day 14

Menu Notes

Food: Portion/Size	Carbohydrate Grams

Breakfast
cheese omelet	2
coffee w/ cream	1
herbal tea	0
	3

Lunch
chicken or tuna salad supreme on bed of lettuce	5
herbal tea	0
	5

Snack
1 oz. cashews	8
1/2 med. apple	10
	18

Dinner
savory pork tenderloin	0
butternut squash salad	6
1 sm. baked potato	20
dry white or red wine	0
	26

Snack
| 1 plum | 6 |
| | Total 58 |

Recipes

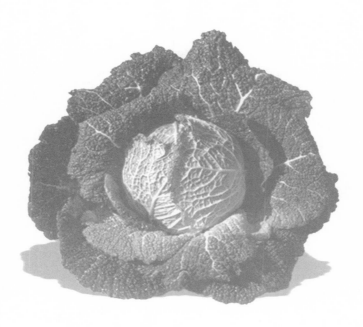

Dressings and Sauces

Portions are measured at grams per serving.

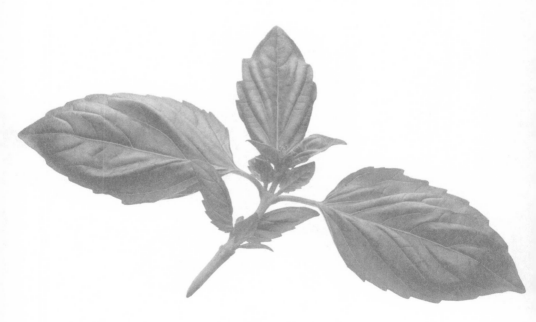

Avocado Dressing: 0.5g

1 med. avocado, chopped
1 med. onion, shredded
1/4 c. picante sauce

1 lg. tomato, chopped
juice of 1 lemon
1/2 c. water

Mix well. Chill.

Balsamic-Basil Herb Dressing: 0g

1/4 c. balsamic vinegar
2 tsp. capers
1/2 tsp. dry mustard
1/2 c. water

1 tsp. dried basil
1 tsp. salt
1/4 c. sunflower oil

Mix in a jar. Shake to blend.

Creamy Red Wine Dressing: 1g

1 c. mayonnaise
1 TBS. dry red wine
1 tsp. McCormick dried salad herbs

4 tsp. prepared horseradish
1/2 tsp. hot sauce

Mix. Refrigerate.

Mar-Na Sauce: 1.5g

1 c. mayonnaise
1 c. cocktail sauce

Mix. Chill.

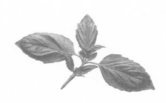

Salads

Portions are measured at grams per serving.

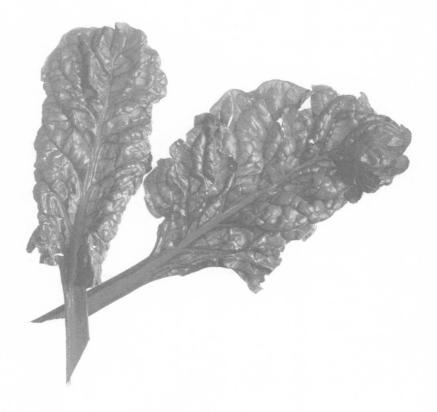

Avocado-Parsley Salad: 8g

1 med. avocado, peeled and chopped
1/4 lb. spinach, washed and torn into bite-sized pieces
1 med. onion, diced
1 bunch parsley, chopped
1/4 c. mild picante sauce
1 lg. tomato, diced
Mix. Chill. Servings: 4

Avocado-Spinach Salad: 7g

1 med. avocado, diced
1/3 bunch fresh basil, chopped
1 med. beet, shredded
1/3 bunch spinach, torn into bite-sized pieces

1 sm. sweet onion, diced
1 med. cucumber, diced

Mix. Chill. Servings: 4

Beet Tops Salad: 4g

tops and stems of 3 beets
1 lg. carrot, shredded
1 yellow pepper, chopped

1 lg. cucumber, chopped
1 med. turnip, shredded
1 stalk celery w/ leaves, chopped

Mix. Chill. Servings: 4

Bok Choy Tomato Salad: 5g

1 bunch bok choy, chopped
1 green pepper, diced
1 stalk celery w/ leaves, chopped
1 med. yellow squash, chopped

1 tomato, diced
1 lg. pickle, diced
1 sm. turnip, shredded
1 sm. carrot, shredded

Mix. Chill. Servings: 4

Butternut Squash Salad: 5g

1 butternut squash, peeled and shredded
1 lg. cucumber, chopped
3 beet tops and stems, chopped
1 med. carrot, shredded   1/4 c. olives, diced
Mix. Chill. Servings: 4

Cabbage-Spinach Salad: 5g

1/4 head of cabbage, chopped   1 med. cucumber, diced
1 sm. zucchini, diced   1 sm. carrot, shredded
1/4 bunch spinach, torn into bite-sized pieces
1 sm. tomato, diced
Mix. Chill. Servings: 4

Cabbage-Turnip Salad: 3.5g

1/4 head white cabbage, chopped   1 sm. turnip, shredded
1 med. carrot, shredded   1 lg. tomato, chopped
1 bunch fresh parsley, chopped
Mix. Chill. Servings: 4

Chef Salad: 5g

1/2 head lettuce
1/2 tomato, chopped
1/2 cucumber, chopped
1 oz. ham, diced
1 oz. chicken, diced
1 oz. cheese, shredded
1 hard-boiled egg, sliced
Mix. Chill. Servings: 4

Chicken Salad Supreme: 5g

2 c. cooked chicken
1 sm. sweet onion, chopped
1/2 tsp. cayenne pepper
1 tsp. celery seed
1/4 c. olives, chopped

1 green pepper, chopped
1 sm. tomato, chopped
1 tsp. salt
1/4 c. mayonnaise

Mix. Chill. Servings: 4

Greek Salad: 6g

1 head romaine lettuce
1/2 onion, diced
1 tomato, chopped
dried herbs: basil, dill, oregano, rosemary

1/2 c. Kalamata olives
1/2 cucumber, chopped
feta cheese

Mix. Chill. Servings: 4

Marina`s Slaw: 8g

1/4 head cabbage, shredded
1 stalk green onion, chopped
1 stalk celery w/ leaves, chopped
1/4 bunch parsley, chopped
1 tsp. lemon juice
1/8 tsp. cayenne pepper

1 sm. turnip, shredded
1 sm. carrot, shredded
1/2 green pepper, chopped
1/4 c. mayonnaise
1 tsp. salt

Mix. Chill. Servings: 4

Mixed Greens-Black Olives Salad: 6g

1/2 lb. mixed greens, washed
1/2 yellow bell pepper, chopped
1/2 c. black Kalamata olives, chopped
1/4 bunch basil, chopped

1 lg. sweet onion, diced
1/2 c. feta cheese

Mix. Chill. Servings: 4

Mixed Greens-Walnut Salad: 7.5g

2 med. tomatoes, diced
1/2 c. English walnuts, chopped
1/4 lb. mixed salad greens, thoroughly washed
1 med. sweet onion, diced
1/4 c. olives, chopped
Mix. Chill. Servings: 4

Mushroom-Pepper Salad: 3g

8 oz. raw mushrooms, chopped
1 med. sweet onion, diced
1/2 bunch parsley, chopped

1 clove garlic, minced

1 red bell pepper, diced
3 tsp. capers
1/4 bunch fresh basil, chopped

Mix. Chill. Serve with blue cheese dressing. Servings: 4

Napa-Beet Salad: 6g

1/2 head Napa
2 stalks celery w/ leaves, chopped
3 med. beets, shredded (save stems and tops)
2 lg. pickles, diced
2 med. tomatoes, chopped
Mix. Chill. Servings: 4

Red Cabbage-Cucumber Salad: 4g

1/2 sm. head red cabbage, chopped
1 med. cucumber, peeled and diced
2 stalks celery w/leaves, chopped
1 spring onion w/ top, chopped
1 sm. zucchini, diced
1 med. carrot, shredded
1/2 c. mild picante sauce
Mix. Chill. Servings: 4

Red Cabbage-Pepper Salad: 5g

1/4 head red cabbage, chopped
1 stalk celery w/ leaves, chopped
1 lg. pickle, chopped
1 green pepper, diced
1 med. carrot, shredded
Mix. Chill. Servings: 4

Red Leaf Lettuce Salad: 8g

1 sm. head red leaf lettuce
1 med. avocado, chopped
1/4 bunch sweet basil, chopped

1 green pepper, chopped
1 med. sweet onion, diced

Mix. Chill. Servings: 4

Romaine-Spinach Salad: 5g

1/3 bunch spinach
10 olives, chopped

1 med. carrot, shredded
1/4 c. almonds

1 sm. bunch romaine lettuce, torn into bite-sized pieces

Mix. Chill. Servings: 4

Tiny Tomato Toss: 4g

1 lb. cherry tomatoes, sliced in half
1 sm. onion, chopped
olive oil

1 sm. cucumber, chopped
1/4 fresh basil, chopped
balsamic vinegar

Mix. Drizzle with oil and vinegar. Servings: 4

Tomato-Cucumber Salad: 6g

2 lg. tomatoes, diced
1 med. sweet onion, diced
few sprigs of parsley, chopped

2 med. cucumbers, diced
1/2 bunch dill, chopped

Mix together. Chill. Drizzle with sunflower oil and balsamic vinegar. Add salt to taste. Servings: 4

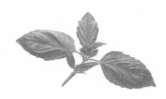

Spreads

Portions are measured at grams per tablespoon

(Use on cabbage leaves, spinach leaves, cucumbers, low-carb crackers.)

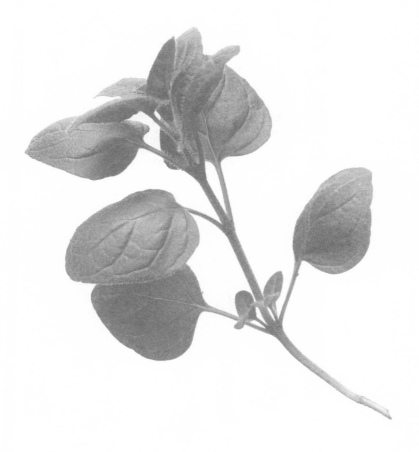

Crab or Tuna Spread: 1.5g

6 oz. crabmeat or white tuna, flaked
8 oz. low-fat cream cheese, softened
cocktail sauce

Spread softened cheese on a plate. Sprinkle fish on top. Cover fish with cocktail sauce. Servings: 6-8

Pecan-Olive Spread: 2g

8 oz. low-fat cream cheese, softened
1 c. pecans, chopped
1/2 c. Kalamata olives (black Greek olives), chopped
1/4 bunch basil, chopped
Mix. Chill. Servings: 6-8

Sun-Dried Tomato-Basil Spread: 0.8g

8 oz. low-fat cream cheese, softened
1/2 jar sun-dried tomatoes packed in oil, chopped
1/4 bunch fresh basil, chopped
Mix. Chill. Servings: 6-8

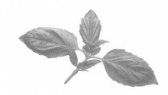

Vegetables

Portions are measured at grams per serving.

(Use the freshest vegetables possible, preferably organically grown.
Slightly steam or sauté them, resulting in a crunchy consistency.)

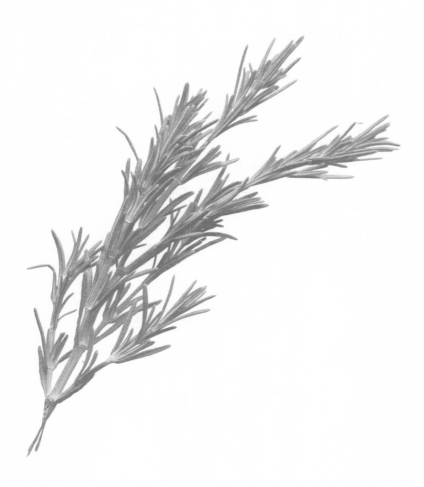

Broccoli with Butter and Garlic: 4g

1 lb. broccoli
2 TBS. sunflower oil
1 tsp. salt
1/2 TBS. granulated garlic
butter

Steam broccoli for 5 minutes. Mix garlic, oil, and salt. Pour over broccoli. Serve with butter. Servings: 4

Broccoli with Picante Sauce: 8g

1 lb. broccoli
1 c. picante sauce
2 TBS. sunflower oil
1 tsp. salt

Steam broccoli until just tender. Mix picante sauce, oil, and salt. Pour over broccoli. Servings: 4

Cheesy-Yellow Squash: 5g

2 lb. sm. yellow squash, sliced lengthwise
cheddar cheese, shredded
3 cloves garlic, chopped

Place squash in a casserole dish. Sprinkle with cheese and 3 garlic. Cover with plastic wrap. Microwave on high for 8 minutes. Servings: 4

Green Beans Almondine: 7g

1 lb. green beans
2 TBS. butter
2 TBS. almonds

Steam beans until just tender. Add butter and almonds. Serve. Servings: 4

Grilled Eggplant: 7g

1 lg. eggplant
1/4 c. olive oil
1/2 tsp. salt

1/2 c. balsamic vinegar
1 clove garlic, minced

Peel eggplant. Slice and soak in salted water for 10 minutes. Squeeze out excess water. Pat dry with paper towels. Mix vinegar, oil, garlic, and salt. Brush mixture onto eggplant. Grill or broil. Servings: 4

Herbed Potatoes: 18g

2 lb. sm. new potatoes, scrubbed and sliced
1 TBS. olive oil   1 tsp. dried thyme

Preheat oven to 350°. Mix ingredients. Place in casserole dish. Cover with foil. Bake 45 minutes. Servings: 4-6

Steamed Cauliflower with Cheese: 5g

1 head cauliflower
1/2 tsp. dried rosemary
1/4 tsp. dried oregano

2 TBS. butter
1/2 tsp. dried basil
shredded cheese

Steam cauliflower until just tender. Add butter and herbs. Sprinkle with shredded cheese. Servings: 4

Tomato-Mushroom Sauté: 8g

1 sm. container mushrooms, chopped
2 lg. tomatoes, chopped
1 tsp. salt
1 tsp. dried basil

1 lg. sweet onion, sliced
3 bay leaves
2 TBS. sunflower oil

Sauté on medium heat until barely cooked (10 min. max.). Servings: 4

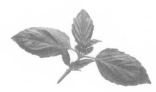

Main Dishes

Portions are measured at grams per serving.

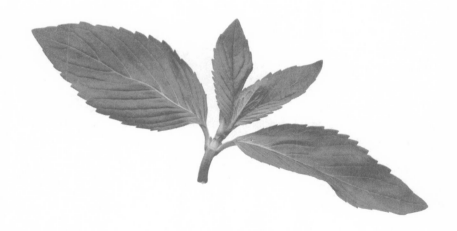

Boiled Shrimp: 2g

2 lb. lg. shrimp
cocktail sauce
salt

Steam shrimp in boiling salted water until they turn white (2-3 min.) Drain. Serve with cocktail sauce. Servings: 4

Broiled Scallops: 0g

2 lb. scallops
dried parsley
lemon juice

celery salt
olive oil
white wine

Preheat oven to 500°. Sprinkle seasonings over scallops. Place in casserole dish. Reduce oven to 400°. Bake scallops 5 minutes. Remove from oven. Sprinkle olive oil over scallops and add 1/2 c. white wine. Cover with foil until served. Servings: 4

Cheese-Onion Omelet: 3g

1 lg. onion-chopped
dried herbs
1/2 C. shredded cheddar cheese
picante sauce

2 TBS. butter
6 eggs
1 clove garlic, minced

Sauté onion in butter. Add herbs and garlic. Beat eggs and Pour over onions. Cover. Cook on medium heat until set. Add 1 TBS. picante sauce per serving. Serves 3-4.

Grilled Scallops: 0g

2 lb. scallops
garlic salt

olive oil
Mar-Na sauce

Preheat oven or grill. Brush scallops with oil. Sprinkle with seasoning. Grill 2 minutes. Turn. Cook 2 additional minutes. Serve with Mar-Na sauce. Servings: 4

Grilled Turkey Patties: 2g

2 lb. ground turkey
1 tsp. garlic powder
1 TBS. dried dill weed

1 lg. onion chopped
1 TBS. dried parsley
1 egg

Combine ingredients. Shape into patties. Grill or broil until centers are no longer pink. Servings: 4-6

Herbed Pork Tenderloin: 0g

2 lb. pork tenderloin
garlic powder

Blackened Redfish Magic
water

Preheat oven to 500°. Sprinkle pork with Redfish Magic and garlic powder. Place in casserole dish. Add 1/2 c. water. Cook 15 minutes. Turn tenderloin. Cook 15 additional min. Add 1/2 c. water. Cover with foil. Reduce heat to 350°. Cook 40 more minutes. Servings: 4-6

Kool Cat Fish Fillets: 0g

2 lb. catfish fillets
Zesty Blend herb seasoning

salt
dry white wine

Preheat oven to 500°. Sprinkle both sides of fillets with herb seasoning and salt. Place in casserole dish. Turn oven to 450°. Bake uncovered until golden brown (15 min.). Turn off oven. Add 1/2 c. dry white wine to dish and cover with foil. Return dish to oven (can remain 2-3 hours). Can also be served cold. Servings: 4

Lemon Caper Turkey: 2g

2 lb. turkey cutlets
capers

olive oil
sliced lemon wedges

Sauté cutlets in oil until center is no longer pink. Arrange on platter and add capers and lemon wedges. Servings: 4

Luscious Leg of Lamb: 2g

1 leg of lamb, cut into pieces
1 lg. onion, sliced
5 bay leaves
2 c. water
salt
garlic powder

Preheat oven to 500°. Season lamb with salt and garlic powder. Cover with onion slices. Add bay leaves and water. Cook uncovered at 500° until brown. Reduce heat to 350°. Add 1 cup water. Cover with foil. Cook 1 additional hour. Servings: 4

Ocean Perch in Tomato-Herb Sauce: 1 lg

2 lb. perch fillets	salt
1 lg. onion, sliced	1/2 c. water
1 lg. carrot, shredded	1 c. tomato sauce
5 bay leaves	10 peppercorns

dried herbs: dill, parsley, thyme, basil, etc.
olive oil

Preheat oven to 350°. Line bottom of pan with sliced onions. Add water. Salt fish. Place on onions. Arrange bay leaves and peppercorns around fish. Sprinkle with herbs. Cover with carrots and then tomato sauce. Cook for 40 minutes. Cover with foil. Return to oven. Sprinkle with oil before serving. Servings: 4

Salmon, Tuna, or Crab Cakes: 4g

1 can salmon or tuna or crab	1 med. onion, chopped
1 egg	1 TBS. dill weed
1 tsp. prepared horseradish	1/4 c. bread crumbs

Combine all ingredients. Shape into patties. Sauté in skillet or grill until golden brown. Servings: 4

Smothered Salmon: 5g

2 lb. salmon
salt
mayonnaise

2 med. onions, sliced
dried dill weed
lemon juice

Preheat oven to 500°. Sprinkle both sides of salmon with salt and dill weed. Place in casserole dish. Cover salmon with onions. Reduce heat to 400°. When onions turn golden brown, cover the dish with foil and cook 10 more minutes. Spread mayonnaise over fish. Sprinkle lemon juice on each serving. Servings: 4

Sassy Soy Chicken Strips: 0g

2 lb. boneless, skinless chicken breast strips
1/4 c. soy sauce
water

Preheat oven to 350°. Place chicken in casserole dish. Add soy sauce and enough water to cover chicken. Cover with foil. Check for doneness after 40-50 min. Cook until browned and tender. Servings: 4

Soy Pork Tenderloin: 0g

2 lb. pork tenderloin
soy sauce
water

Preheat oven to 500°. Sprinkle pork with soy sauce. Place in casserole dish. Add 1 c. water. Cover with foil. Bake 1 1/2 hours. Servings: 4

Tender Baked Chicken: 0g

6 lb. baking hen
garlic powder
Vege-Sal seasoning or soy sauce

Preheat oven to 500°. Cut chicken in half. Place in drip baking pan. Sprinkle with seasonings. Cover with foil. Bake 30 min. then reduce heat to 350°. Bake 2-4 additional hours. Servings: 4

Terrific Trout: 2g

2 lb. steelhead trout

dried parsley

lemon juice

olive oil

salt

cayenne pepper

2 TBS. capers

Preheat oven to 500°. Sprinkle both sides of fish with salt and herbs. Place in casserole dish. Reduce heat to 400°. Bake uncovered 7-10 minutes. Turn off heat. Sprinkle water and olive oil over fish. Add capers. Cover with foil. Return to oven. Servings: 4

Tofu for You!: less than 1g

1 box extra firm organic tofu

1 lb. asparagus spears

sesame seeds (opt.)

soy sauce

water

Slice tofu lengthwise into 4 servings. Sauté in soy sauce. Add asparagus, more soy sauce, and water. Cook 3-4 min. Sprinkle with sesame seeds if desired. Servings: 4

Western Omelet: 3g

2 eggs, beaten

2 TBS. onion, diced

1/4 green pepper, chopped

ham and cheese, diced

Sauté onion and pepper in butter until soft. Add eggs. Cover. Cook until set. Sprinkle with ham and cheese. Servings: 1-2

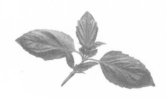

Carbohydrate Counter

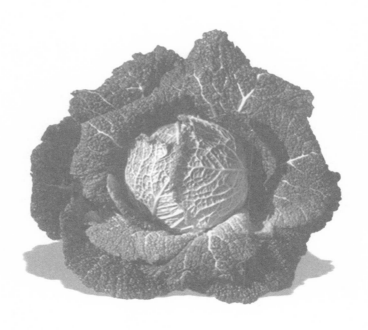

Food	Portion/Size	Grams
A		
Alfalfa seeds, sprouted	1 c.	1.2
Almonds	1/2 c.	10
Apple, raw	1/2 med.	10
Apricot, raw	1	4
Apricot, dried halves	1 c.	80.3
Asparagus, fresh	1 lb.	12.7
Avocado, raw	1 lb.	8.9
Avocado puree	1/2 c.	8.5
B		
Bacon	2 strips	trace
Bacon, Canadian	3-4 slices	trace
Bagel, egg	3"	28.3
Bagel, regular	3"	30
Bagel, cinnamon-raisin	3 1/8 oz.	36
Bagel, onion	1	30
Bagel chips	1 oz.	20
Banana	lg.	30.2

Food	Portion/Size	Grams
Banana, mashed	1 c.	50
Barley, pearl, cooked	1 c.	44.3
Bass, raw	any size	0
Beans, baked w/ tomato sauce	1 c.	58.8
Beans, canned black or brown	1 c.	42
Beans, fresh green	1 lb.	28.3
Beans, boiled green	1/2 c.	3.3
Beans, kidney or red	1/2 c.	19.8
Beans, pinto	1/2 c.	18
Beans, refried	1/2 c.	15
Beef, canned/dried/chipped	any size	0
Beef	any size	0
Beef, roast	any size	0
Beef, round steak	any size	0
Beef, other	any size	0
Beer, Anheuser	12 oz.	15.4
Beer, Coors	12 oz.	11.4
Beer, Budweiser Light	12 oz.	6.7
Beer, Michelob Light	12 oz.	11.5

Food	Portion/Size	Grams
Beer, Rolling Rock	12 oz.	8
Beets, raw	1 lb.	31.4
Beets, diced	1/2 c.	6.6
Biscuits, Big Premium Heat 'n Eat	1	16
Biscuits, Cinnamon Raisin Grands	1	27
Biscuits, Hungry Jack Extra Rich	1	9
Biscuits, oat bran/honey nut	1	19
Biscuits, white/regular	1	16
Blackberries, raw	1/2 c.	10
Blueberries, raw	1/2 c.	11
Bologna	1 slice	1
Bran, crude	1 oz.	17.5
Bran, miller's	1 TBS.	2.8
Brandy	any size	0
Brazil nuts, shelled	1/2 c.	7.5
Bread, 5 Bran	1 slice	13
Bread, Cinnamon	1 slice	15
Bread, Sweetheart French	1 slice	14

Food	Portion/Size	Grams
Bread, Country Farms Mountain oat	1 slice	23
Bread, Brannola	1 slice	14
Bread, honey oat bran	1 slice	12.7
Bread, oatmeal	1 slice	17
Bread, Pritikin onion dill	1 slice	12
Bread, pita white	1 slice	31
Bread, pita whole wheat	1 slice	28
Bread, pumpernickel	1 slice	14
Bread, Arnold Tea Raisin	1 slice	13
Bread, Jewish rye	1 slice	14
Bread, stone ground whole wheat	1 slice	8
Bread, Little Caesar's Crazy	1 piece	18
Broccoli, raw	1 c.	7
Burrito, bean and cheese	5 oz.	46.9
Burrito, breakfast w/egg, bacon, cheese	1	27.9
Burrito, breakfast hot and spicy	1	30

Food	Portion/Size	Grams

C

Food	Portion/Size	Grams
Cabbage, raw	1 lb.	19.3
Cabbage, raw	1 c.	4.9
Cantaloupe, cubed	1/2 c.	6.1
Carrots, raw, diced	1/2 c.	7
Cashews	1/4 c.	7.5
Catsup, regular	1 TBS.	4
Cauliflower, raw	1 c.	5
Caviar	1 oz.	1.1
Celery	1 stalk	1.6
Cheese, American	1 oz.	0.6
Cheese, blue	1 oz.	0.6
Cheese, cheddar	1 oz.	0.6
Cheese, cottage	1 c.	4.5
Cheese, cream	1 TBS.	0.3
Cheese, edam	1 oz.	1.1
Cheese, feta	1 oz.	0.5
Cheese, gruyere	1 oz.	0.5
Cheese, grated parmesan	1 TBS.	0.2

Food	Portion/Size	Grams
Cheese, provolone	1 oz.	0.8
Cheese, Swiss	1 oz.	0.5
Cheese, Velveeta	1 oz.	3
Cheese spreads, bacon, olive, etc.	1 oz.	1.9
Cherry, sweet, fresh, whole	1/2 c.	10.2
Chicken	any size	0
Chick-Peas or garbanzo beans, cooked	1/2 c.	22
Coconut, fresh, grated	1/2 c.	6.1
Corn, boiled	1 ear	16.2
Crab salad	1/2 c.	30
Crackers, cheese	27	16
Crackers, Ritz	5	10
Crackers, saltines	5	10
Crackers, Triscuits	7	21
Crackers, Wasa Rye	2	10
Crackers, Wheat Thins	17	21
Cranberries, fresh	1/2 c.	6
Cranberry, Ocean Spray Juice Cocktail	6 oz.	25.4

Food	Portion/Size	Grams
Cream, heavy	1 TBS.	0.5
Cream, sour	1 TBS.	0.5
Cucumber	1 lg.	7

D

Dates, dry, domestic, without pits	4 oz.	82.7
Dip, onion w/ sour cream	1 TBS.	1.5
Dip, seafood w/ sour cream	1 TBS.	0.4
Deviled eggs	1	0.5
Drambuie, 80 proof	1 oz.	11
Duck	any size	0
Dunkin' Donuts, chocolate croissant	1	38
Dunkin' Donuts, filled jelly donut	1	31
Dunkin' Donuts, glazed buttermilk donut	1	37
Dunkin' Donuts, glazed yeast donut	1	26
Dunkin' Donuts, bran muffin w/ raisins	1	51

Food	Portion/Size	Grams

E

Eggplant, raw	1 lb.	20.6
Eggplant, boiled/drained/diced	1 c.	8.2
Endive, curly/raw/untrimmed	1 lb.	16.4
Endive, shredded	1 c.	2.9
Espresso coffee liqueur, 26 1/2% alcohol	1 oz	15

F

Fajitas, Healthy Choice	7 oz. meal	26
Fajitas, beef	6 3/4 oz. meal	31
Fettuccini, Weight Watchers Alfredo	8 oz. meal	28
Fig, fresh	1.3 oz	7.7
Fish	any size	0
Fish fillet, lightly breaded	1	16
French toast, Aunt Jemima regular	5.9 oz. meal	53

Food	Portion/Size	Grams

G

Gin	any size	0
Gefilte Fish	2 oz.	4.8
Goose	any size	0
Granola bar, oat bran honey graham	0.8 oz.	16
Granola bar, cookies and creme	1.2 oz.	23
Granola cereal, cinnamon and raisin, fruit and nut	1/3 c.	19
Granola cereal, raisins and dates	1/4 c.	20
Granola snack, chocolate chip	1.25 oz.	21
Granola snack, cinnamon or honey nut	1 pouch	19
Grapes	1 c.	15
Grape Nuts cereal	1/4 c.	23
Grapefruit	1/2 sm.	10
Gravy, La Choy brown	2 oz.	4.4
Guava	1	11.7
Gum	1 stick	1.7
Gum, candy-coated	1 stick	1.3

Food	Portion/Size	Grams

H

Food	Portion/Size	Grams
Ham	any size	0
Hamburger, plain	1 c.	9
Hamburger, McDonald's plain with bun	3.6 oz.	34
Hazelnuts, Filberts,	10-12	5
Herring, raw, pickled, smoked	any size	0
Honey, strained	1 TBS.	16.5
Honeydew melon	1 med. wedge	8

I

Food	Portion/Size	Grams
Ice-cream	1/2 c.	15

J

Food	Portion/Size	Grams
Jelly, Empress Grape	1 TBS.	13.5

K

Food	Portion/Size	Grams
Kiwi	1 med.	11

Food	Portion/Size	Grams

L

Lamb	any size	0
Lasagna w/ meat sauce	12 oz.	38
Lasagna, mix	1/5 of pkg.	33
Lasagna, pizza dish	1/5 of pkg.	37
Lasagna, Sorrentino cheese,	8 oz.	37.4
Lasagna, Celentano, Great Choice, low-fat	10 oz.	42
Leeks, raw, trimmed	4 oz.	12.7
Lemons, peeled	2 1/8"	6.1
Lemon juice	1 TBS.	1.2
Lentils, cooked, drained	1/2 c.	19.5
Lettuce, Iceberg, untrimmed	1 lb.	8.4
Lime juice	1 TBS.	0.5
Linguini, canned w/ clam sauce	1 serving	30
Linguini, Healthy Balance	11 1/2 oz. meal	49
Litchi nut, flesh only	4 oz.	18.6
Liver, chicken	3 oz.	3
Lobster, cocktail	1 c., cooked	1.9

Food	Portion/Size	Grams

M

Macadamia nuts	1 oz.	4.5
Macaroni, cooked	4 oz.	26
Mango, fresh, diced or sliced	1/2 c.	13.8
Manicotti, frozen	9 oz.	45
Mayonnaise	1 TBS.	0
Meatballs, cocktail	any size	0
Meatballs, Swedish, frozen w/ noodles	10 oz. meal	37
Meat loaf dinner, frozen, low-fat/low-cholesterol	12 oz.	48
Mayonnaise	1 TBS.	trace
Mexican frozen dinner, Banquet combination	12 oz. meal	72
Mexican frozen dinner, Patio, regular	13 1/4 oz. meal	64
Mexican frozen dinner, Swanson Hungry Man	20 1/4 oz meal	88
Milk, low-fat buttermilk	1 c.	12
Milk, low-fat chocolate	1 c.	29
Milk, whole	1 c.	12
Milk, skim	8 oz.	12

Food	Portion/Size	Grams
Milk, soy bean,	1/2 c	1.5
Molasses	1 TBS.	13.3
Muesli, cereal w/ raisins, dates, almonds	1/2 c.	32
Muffins	1	20-50
Mushrooms	1/2 c.	4.4
Mussels, smoked	1	trace

N

Nectarines, raw	1 med.	8
Noodles, dry	1 oz.	20.4
Noodles and Chicken, frozen dinner	10 oz.	42
Nuts, mixed	8-12	2.7

O

Oatmeal, dry, regular	1/2 c.	44.5
Okra, boiled, whole	1/2 c.	5.3
Olives, green	5 lg.	0.5
Olives, black	5 lg.	1
Onions, raw, whole	2 1/2"	8.7

Food	Portion/Size	Grams
Oranges, fresh	2 4/5"	15.5
Oysters, raw	3-4 med.	4
Oysters, smoked	4-6 sm.	2.6

P

Food	Portion/Size	Grams
Pancakes, frozen, buttermilk	1	17
Papayas, fresh, cubed	1 c.	18.2
Parsley	1 TBS.	0.3
Parsnips, cooked	1/2 c.	15.8
Pâté de foie gras	1 TBS.	0.7
Peas, green, shelled	1/2 c.	9.9
Peaches	1 med.	9
Peanut butter, natural	1 TBS.	3.5
Pears, fresh, whole	3"	25.4
Pecans, halves	1/2 c.	7.9
Peppers, green	1 med.	3
Peppers, red	1 med.	5
Pickles, dill	1 lg.	2
Pies	all varieties	50-74

Food	Portion/Size	Grams
Pineapples, fresh, diced	1/2 c.	10.7
Pistachio nuts	20	1.6
Pizza, Little Caesar's Baby Pan! Pan!	1 whole	53
Pizza, cheese and pepperoni	1 slice	16
Pizza, Pizza Hut cheese	1	27
Pizza, Pizza Hut Personal Pan pepperoni	1	76
Pizza, Pizza Hut Personal Pan supreme	1	76
Plums	1	6
Popcorn, popped	1 c.	10
Pop Tarts	1	32
Potatoes, sweet	1 sm.	38.5
Potatoes, baked	1/2 c.	16
Pretzels	5	4
Prunes, stewed	1/2 c	32
Prunes, dried	2 oz	31

Food	Portion/Size	Grams

R

Radishes	8 sm.	2
Raisins	1/2 c	62.7
Raspberries, red	1/2 c.	9
Rhubarb, cubed, sweetened	1/2 c	43.2
Rice, cooked, brown	2/3 c	26.4
Rice, cooked, white	2/3 c	22.5
Rice cake	1	9
Rum	any size	0

S

Salad dressing, Blue cheese	1 TBS.	1.1
Salad dressing, Buttermilk	1 TBS.	0
Salad dressing, Caesar	1 TBS.	1
Salad dressing, French	1 TBS.	.6
Salad dressing, Italian	1 TBS.	1
Salad dressing, Ranch	1 TBS.	2
Salad dressing, Russian	1 TBS.	1.6
Salad dressing, Thousand Island	1 TBS.	2.5

Food	Portion/Size	Grams
Salmon	any size	0
Salmon, canned	any size	0
Sandwich spread	1 TBS.	2.4
Sandwiches, ham and cheese	1	55
Sandwiches, tuna melt	1	58
Sardines, canned	any size	0
Sausage, pork	8 oz.	trace
Sausage, Polish	4 oz.	1.3
Scallops	0	
Schnapps	1 oz	7.5
Scotch whiskey	any size	0
Sesame seeds	1 oz	5
Shrimp	4 lg.	trace
Sirloin	any size	0
Soft drinks, diet	12 oz.	trace
Soft drinks, Coca Cola	12 oz.	40
Soft drinks, Dr. Pepper	12 oz.	38.9
Soft drinks, Ginger Ale	12 oz.	31.6
Soft drinks, Minute Maid Orange	12 oz.	44

Food	Portion/Size	Grams
Soft drinks, Pepsi	12 oz.	39
Soft drinks, RC 100	12 oz.	42.8
Soft drinks, root beer	12 oz.	42
Soft drinks, Fanta	12 oz.	40
Soft drinks, 7 Up	12 oz.	36.2
Soft drinks, Sprite	12 oz.	36
Sorbet, Baskin Robins orange	1/2 c	29.7
Sorbet, Baskin Robins raspberry	1/2 c	34
Soy beans, cooked	1/2 c	8.4
Soy bean curd/Tofu	4 oz	2.7
Soy sauce	1 TBS.	1
Spinach, raw	3 1/2 oz.	4
Sports drink, any flavor	16 oz.	28
Squash, summer, cooked	1/2 c.	4
Sunflower seeds	1 oz	5.6
Strawberries, raw	1 c.	10
Syrup, Aunt Jemima	1 TBS.	7.3
Syrup, corn, karo	1 TBS.	14.5
Syrup, maple	1 TBS.	13

Food	Portion/Size	Grams
Syrup, Mrs. Butterworth	1 TBS.	7.5
Syrup, Weight Watchers	1 TBS.	6

T

Food	Portion/Size	Grams
Tabbouleh mix	1/2 c	20
Tacos, Old El Paso shell	1	6
Tacos, Taco Bell regular	1	10.6
Taco salad, Taco Bell	1	26.3
Taco sauce, Taco Bell	1 pkg.	.4
Tangerines	1 med.	10
Tapioca, dry	1 TBS.	7.9
Tea, herbal, unsweetened	1 c.	0.4
Tea, unsweetened	8 oz.	trace
Teriyaki sauce	1 TBS.	.6
Textured Vegetable Protein, Morningstar Farms breakfast links	1	1.3
Textured Vegetable Protein, Morningstar Farms breakfast patties	1	3.4
Textured Vegetable Protein, Morningstar Farms breakfast strips	1	.6

Food	Portion/Size	Grams
Textured Vegetable Protein, Morningstar Farms breakfast grillers	1	6
Tomatoes, raw	1 sm.	4
Tomato paste, canned, regular	6 oz	35
Tomato sauce, canned, regular	1/2 c	8
Tomatoes, sun-dried in oils w/ herbs	1 oz	9
Toppings, Smuckers butterscotch	1 TBS.	16.5
Toppings, Smuckers caramel	1 TBS.	14
Toppings, Hershey's fudge	1 TBS.	9
Toppings, Smuckers marshmallow	1 TBS.	14.5
Toppings, Cool Whip	1 TBS.	1.2
Tortillas, corn	1	10
Tortillas, flour	1	27
Tostadas, Old El Paso shell	1	6
Trout	any size	0
Tuna, canned	any size	0
Tuna salad	1/2 c.	2.5
Turkey	any size	0
Turkey pie, regular	7 oz	39

Food	Portion/Size	Grams
Turnips, fresh, w/ skins	1 lb.	25.7
Turnips, paired, untrimmed	1/2 lb.	4.4
Turnip greens, fresh	1 lb.	19
Turnip greens, boiled	1/2 lb.	2.6
Twinkies, banana-golden-cream filled	1	27
Twinkies, light	1	21

U

Ultra Slim Fast, canned, French vanilla	12 oz.	38
Ultra Slim Fast, regular, cafe mocha	8 oz.	38
Ultra Slim Fast, plus, chocolate fantasy	12 oz.	50
Ultra Slim Fast, pina colada mix w/ fruit juices	8 oz.	43

V

Veal	any size	0
Vegetable juice, Knudsen and Sons veggie, regular, spicy	6 oz.	6
Vienna sausage	3 1/2 oz.	3
Vinegar, balsamic	1 TBS.	2

Food	Portion/Size	Grams
Vinegar, cider	1 TBS.	.9
Vodka	any size	0

W

Waffle, frozen (Egg o)	1	16
Walnuts, English	1/2 c.	8
Water chestnuts, peeled	4 oz	21.5
Watercress, raw, untrimmed	1/2 c	.5
Watermelon	1/2 c.	5.1
Wheat germ, raw	1 TBS.	3.2
Wine coolers, Bartles and Jaymes, berry	6 oz.	16
Wine coolers, tropical	6 oz.	18.5
Wine coolers, light: berry	6 oz.	16
Wine coolers, tropical	6 oz.	16.5
Wine, dry red or white	4 oz.	0.5
Wonton Wrapper, Nasoya	1 pc.	20

Food	Portion/Size	Grams

Y

Food	Portion/Size	Grams
Yogurt, TCBY, 96% fat free	8.2 oz	47
Yogurt, TCBY, regular fat free	8.2 oz	47
Yogurt, TCBY, regular fat free/sugar free	8.2 oz	37
Yogurt, Breyers, strawberry	8 oz.	46
Yogurt shake, Weight Watchers, chocolate	7.5 oz	44

Z

Food	Portion/Size	Grams
Zingers (Dolly Madison), chocolate	1 pc.	23
Zweiback, Nabisco	1 pc.	5

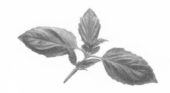

Personal Menu

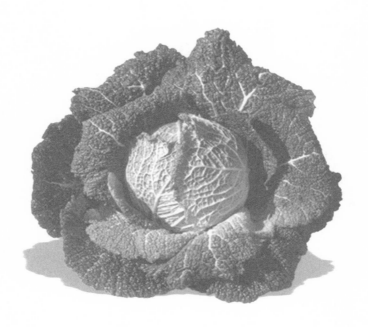

Breakfast:

....

....

....

Total Carbohydrates:

....

Lunch:

....

....

....

Total Carbohydrates:

....

Snack:

....

Total Carbohydrates:

....

Dinner:

....

....

....

Total Carbohydrates:

....

Snack:

....

....

Total Carbohydrates:

....

Breakfast:

Total Carbohydrates:

Lunch:

Total Carbohydrates:

Snack:

Total Carbohydrates:

Dinner:

Total Carbohydrates:

Snack:

Total Carbohydrates:

Breakfast:

....

....

....

Total Carbohydrates:

Lunch:

....

....

....

Total Carbohydrates:

Snack:

....

Total Carbohydrates:

Dinner:

....

....

....

Total Carbohydrates:

Snack:

....

Total Carbohydrates:

Breakfast:

....

....

....

Total Carbohydrates:

....

Lunch:

....

....

....

Total Carbohydrates:

....

Snack:

....

Total Carbohydrates:

....

Dinner:

....

....

....

Total Carbohydrates:

....

Snack:

....

Total Carbohydrates:

....

Personal Menus - Day 5

Breakfast:

....

....

....

Total Carbohydrates:
....

Lunch:

....

....

....

Total Carbohydrates:
....

Snack:

....

Total Carbohydrates:
....

Dinner:

....

....

....

Total Carbohydrates:
....

Snack:

....

Total Carbohydrates:
....

Breakfast:

....

....

Total Carbohydrates:
....

Lunch:

....

Total Carbohydrates:
....

Snack:
....

Total Carbohydrates:
....

Dinner:

....

....

Total Carbohydrates:
....

Snack:
....

Total Carbohydrates:
....

Breakfast:

Total Carbohydrates:

Lunch:

Total Carbohydrates:

Snack:

Total Carbohydrates:

Dinner:

Total Carbohydrates:

Snack:

Total Carbohydrates:

Breakfast:

....

....

Total Carbohydrates:

Lunch:

....

....

Total Carbohydrates:

Snack:

....

Total Carbohydrates:

Dinner:

....

....

....

Total Carbohydrates:

Snack:

....

Total Carbohydrates:

Breakfast:

Total Carbohydrates:

Lunch:

Total Carbohydrates:

Snack:

Total Carbohydrates:

Dinner:

Total Carbohydrates:

Snack:

Total Carbohydrates:

Breakfast:

Total Carbohydrates:

Lunch:

Total Carbohydrates:

Snack:

Total Carbohydrates:

Dinner:

Total Carbohydrates:

Snack:

Total Carbohydrates:

Breakfast:

....

....

....

Total Carbohydrates:

Lunch:

....

....

Total Carbohydrates:

Snack:

....

Total Carbohydrates:

Dinner:

....

....

....

Total Carbohydrates:

Snack:

....

Total Carbohydrates:

Breakfast:

....

....

....

....   Total Carbohydrates:

Lunch:

....

....

....   Total Carbohydrates:

Snack:

....

....   Total Carbohydrates:

Dinner:

....

....

....

....   Total Carbohydrates:

Snack:

....

....   Total Carbohydrates:

Breakfast:

Total Carbohydrates:

Lunch:

Total Carbohydrates:

Snack:

Total Carbohydrates:

Dinner:

Total Carbohydrates:

Snack:

Total Carbohydrates:

Breakfast:

....

....

....

Total Carbohydrates:
....

Lunch:

....

....

....

Total Carbohydrates:
....

Snack:

....

....

Total Carbohydrates:
....

Dinner:

....

....

....

....

Total Carbohydrates:
....

Snack:

....

....

Total Carbohydrates:
....

Works Cited

Balch, James F., and Phyllis A. *Prescription for Cooking and Dietary Wellness*. Greenfield, IN: P.A.B. Publishing, 1992.

Gittleman, Ann Louise. *Get the Sugar Out!* New York: Three Rivers Press, 1996.

Loiselle, Beth. *The Healing Power of Whole Foods*. Nicholasville, KY: Healthways Nutrition, 1993.

Sears, Barry. *Zone-Perfect Meals in Minutes*. New York: HarperCollins, 1997.

Wade, Carlson. *Health Secrets from the Orient*. West Nyack, NY: Parker Publishing, 1973.